# Pocket Flow Charts for Symptom Control

by Peter Kaye

MA MB BCh FRCP MRCGP
Consultant in Palliative Medicine

# CONTENTS

This book uses clear flow charts to highlight important questions for controlling common symptoms in palliative care.

It is especially for busy GPs and hospital doctors who want clear simple management pathways.

The flow charts are extracted from a longer (223 page) book called "Decision Making in Palliative Care" by Peter Kaye (see inside back cover) which includes many other flow charts covering:

- Other less common physical symptoms
- Psychological, psycho-social and family problems
- Organisational and ethical dilemmas
- Developing clinical guidelines

Peter Kaye

# ANALGESICS

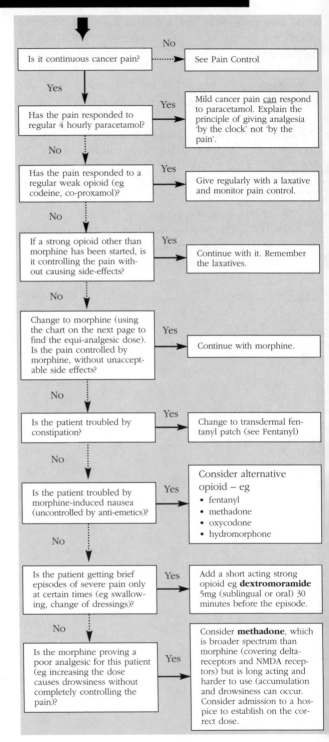

Is it continuous cancer pain? —— No ·······▶ See Pain Control

Yes ↓

Has the pain responded to regular 4 hourly paracetamol? —— Yes ▶ Mild cancer pain <u>can</u> respond to paracetamol. Explain the principle of giving analgesia 'by the clock' not 'by the pain'.

No ↓

Has the pain responded to a regular weak opioid (eg codeine, co-proxamol)? —— Yes ▶ Give regularly with a laxative and monitor pain control.

No ↓

If a strong opioid other than morphine has been started, is it controlling the pain without causing side-effects? —— Yes ▶ Continue with it. Remember the laxatives.

No ↓

Change to morphine (using the chart on the next page to find the equi-analgesic dose). Is the pain controlled by morphine, without unacceptable side effects? —— Yes ▶ Continue with morphine.

No ↓

Is the patient troubled by constipation? —— Yes ▶ Change to transdermal fentanyl patch (see Fentanyl)

No ↓

Is the patient troubled by morphine-induced nausea (uncontrolled by anti-emetics)? —— Yes ▶ Consider alternative opioid – eg
• fentanyl
• methadone
• oxycodone
• hydromorphone

No ↓

Is the patient getting brief episodes of severe pain only at certain times (eg swallowing, change of dressings)? —— Yes ▶ Add a short acting strong opioid eg **dextromoramide** 5mg (sublingual or oral) 30 minutes before the episode.

No ↓

Is the morphine proving a poor analgesic for this patient (eg increasing the dose causes drowsiness without completely controlling the pain)? —— Yes ▶ Consider **methadone**, which is broader spectrum than morphine (covering delta-receptors and NMDA receptors) but is long acting and harder to use (accumulation and drowsiness can occur. Consider admission to a hospice to establish on the correct dose.

## Is it a constant pain?

This section is about the use of analgesics for <u>constant</u> aching pain. (For intermittent pains, see Pain Control). If a patient is getting a constant aching pain they need regular analgesia. Teach them to take it "by the clock, not by the pain" and write out a drug card for them.

## Has the patient already tried any analgesics?

The analgesic history can give you helpful clues about how to manage the pain. For example if the patient has tried taking two Solpadol tablets (which contains 30mg codeine plus 500mg paracetamol – like Tylex and Kapake) and noticed that the pain went for 2 hours and then returned, it guides you. It means that 60mg codeine is giving only 2 hours pain control, therefore the patient needs to start a stronger regular analgesic, eg morphine 5mg 4 hourly, or a 25mcg\hr fentanyl patch.

## What is the "analgesic ladder"?

The analgesic ladder is simply a common-sense approach to choosing an appropriate analgesic for the severity of pain, eg:
- mild pain – paracetamol
- moderate pain – codeine
- severe pain – morphine or fentanyl

## How do you select the right analgesic?

Pain is invisible so you have to be guided by the patient's description, plus the response to analgesics already tried, plus the patient's behaviour – eg a patient lying still and sweating and groaning with pain would be started on Diamorphine 2–5mg IM rather than paracetamol.

## Is morphine the best analgesic for severe cancer pain?

Morphine has been considered the best strong analgesic for continuous cancer pain with the advantages of a short half-life (2.5 hours) and no maximum dose, but other opioid analgesics can have advantages, eg:
- fentanyl – fewer side-effects
- methadone – broader spectrum and safe in renal failure
- dextromoramide – short-term boost in analgesia.

# ASCITES

**Are you sure the distension is due to ascites?**
→ No → Ultrasound scan will confirm (?aspirate under ultrasound if loculated).

↓ Yes

**Is it causing any problems?**
→ No → Explain cause and treatment options to patient. Explain it is likely to worsen.

↓ Yes

**Is oncology treatment still an option?**
→ Yes → Ascites can respond to chemotherapy. For example even in advanced carcinoma of the ovary, oral chlorambucil can reduce ascites.

↓ No

**Is prognosis short (hours or days)?**
→ Yes → The best option may be to treat symptoms and leave the ascites alone.

↓ No

**Is paracentesis possible?**
→ Yes → (ie No gross bowel distension, adhesions or tumour masses.) Drain up to 5L. If hypotension occurs consider IV albumin. Consider starting diuretics which may delay recurrence.

↓ No

**Can the patient tolerate diuretics?**
→ Yes → Patients with a lot of oedema may tolerate high doses of diuretics (Frusemide 80mg BD and Spironolactone 400 mg BD) for a limited period. Consider a short-term indwelling catheter. Monitor U&Es and girth measurement and reduce diuretic dose as appropriate.

↓ No

**Is a P-V shunt appropriate (and patient agrees)?**
→ Yes → Consider an early P-V shunt if prognosis is still in months. Refer to surgeon (unless there is a bleeding tendency, or thick blood in the fluid). A shunt can give good palliation for several months.

↓ No

Continue to treat any **symptoms** caused by the ascites:
- dyspnoea
- pain
- dyspepsia
- hiccups
- nausea

## Is the distension due to ascites (fluid)?

Abdominal distension may be due to tumour, bowel destruction, a very large liver or ascites (which simply means free fluid in the abdominal cavity). Free fluid causes the physical side of "shifting dullness". If in doubt, ultrasound scan is very helpful.

## Is the ascites due to cancer?

In advance cancer abdominal ascites is almost always malignant, but it is worth remembering that there are other causes of ascites (cirrhosis, tuberculosis).

## Has it been "tapped" before?

If the fluid has already been successfully drained by paracentesis it is usually an easy procedure to repeat the drainage if necessary. However it there is uncertainty that the abdominal distension is due to ascites (or whether the ascites is locculated), ultra sound scan should be considered before a first paracentesis.

## Is it causing symptoms?

Symptoms include discomfort and difficulty bending, dyspnoea and gastric reflux (dyspepsia, hiccups, nausea). Secondary leg oedema can occur. One option may be to treat the secondary symptoms and leave the ascites alone, especially in a patient with a short prognosis.

## Does the patient need urgent relief?

The quickest way of providing relief is parcentesis.

## Can the patient tolerate high dose diuretics?

A combination of Frusimide 80mg daily and Spironolactone 200mg daily can slow down the recurrence of malignant ascites, especially after a paracentesis. This is useful treatment if the patient not only has ascites but also leg oedema. But the diuretics may cause unacceptable urinary frequency (and spironolactone can cause nausea.) If high dose diuretics are started monitor (U and E levels and abdominal girth measurements.) Reduce the dose once the ascites has resolved otherwise the patient can become dehydrated.

## Is the fluid white and milky?

White milky fluid is called "chylous" and is due to a leak of lymphatic fluid from the thoracic duct, usually because it has been invaded by carcinoma. It is very difficult to manage, it tends to recur quickly after paracentesis and does not respond to diuretics, and the fluid is too thick usually to consider a PV shunt. Usually it is a pre-terminal event.

## Does the patient need a shunt?

A peritoneo-venous shunt can be a very effective way of managing ascites, particularly in patients with a long prognosis (to avoid the need of repeated paracentesis.) A shunt can be inserted under local anaesthetic but is usually preferably done under general anaesthetic. It is contra-indicated if the patient is anti-coagulated or if the fluid is thick or blood stained fluid. A shunt can last many months. 30% of them eventually block and may need replacing.

# BLEEDING

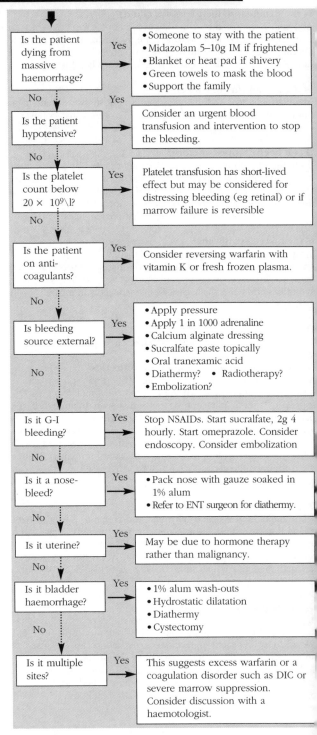

| | | |
|---|---|---|
| Is the patient dying from massive haemorrhage? | Yes | • Someone to stay with the patient<br>• Midazolam 5–10g IM if frightened<br>• Blanket or heat pad if shivery<br>• Green towels to mask the blood<br>• Support the family |
| Is the patient hypotensive? | Yes | Consider an urgent blood transfusion and intervention to stop the bleeding. |
| Is the platelet count below $20 \times 10^9 \backslash l$? | Yes | Platelet transfusion has short-lived effect but may be considered for distressing bleeding (eg retinal) or if marrow failure is reversible |
| Is the patient on anti-coagulants? | Yes | Consider reversing warfarin with vitamin K or fresh frozen plasma. |
| Is bleeding source external? | Yes | • Apply pressure<br>• Apply 1 in 1000 adrenaline<br>• Calcium alginate dressing<br>• Sucralfate paste topically<br>• Oral tranexamic acid<br>• Diathermy? • Radiotherapy?<br>• Embolization? |
| Is it G-I bleeding? | Yes | Stop NSAIDs. Start sucralfate, 2g 4 hourly. Start omeprazole. Consider endoscopy. Consider embolization |
| Is it a nose-bleed? | Yes | • Pack nose with gauze soaked in 1% alum<br>• Refer to ENT surgeon for diathermy. |
| Is it uterine? | Yes | May be due to hormone therapy rather than malignancy. |
| Is it bladder haemorrhage? | Yes | • 1% alum wash-outs<br>• Hydrostatic dilatation<br>• Diathermy<br>• Cystectomy |
| Is it multiple sites? | Yes | This suggests excess warfarin or a coagulation disorder such as DIC or severe marrow suppression. Consider discussion with a haemotologist. |

## Can the bleeding be controlled?

There are a number of ways of controlling bleeding (that are often overlooked). Tranexamic acid can be very effective, other methods are described in the flow chart opposite.

## Is the patient frightened?

Even very minor bleeding terrifies some patients who see it as life threatening. A bit of explanation can be very therapeutic.

## Is oral iron indicated?

Long-term low-grade bleeding such as haematuria depletes iron stores and the patient should be on oral iron supplements.

## Is a blood transfusion indicated?

Blood transfusion is only indicated if the bleeding has been controlled, otherwise it simply worsens the haemorrhage.

## Is radiotherapy indicated?

Radiotherapy can effectively control haemorrhage and should always be considered in tumours of the lung, bladder, uterus, vagina or rectum.

## Is platelet transfusion indicated?

Marrow involvement that has reduced the platelet count to below $10 \times 10^9 \backslash l$ causes spontaneous haemorrhages (purpura or bruising may be visible). Platelet transfusion is only effective in controlling bleeding for 2 or 3 days but may be indicated even in the terminal phase if the effects of bleeding is particularly devastating (eg retinal haemorrhages).

## Is heavy terminal bleeding likely?

A patient who has invasion of a major artery such as carotid or femoral and has had some warning bleeds may die from massive haemorrhage. Have green towels available (which reduce the impact of red blood on white sheets) and if it happens someone should stay with the patient. Somebody else should draw up diamorphine and midazolam but should ask the patient before giving it. If masive haemorrhage is a very strong possibility the timing of explanation and fore-warning to both the patient and family is a matter of judgement.

# CONFUSION

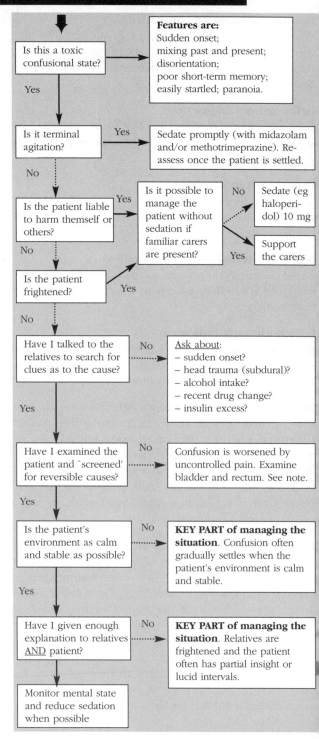

**Is this a toxic confusional state?** → **Features are:** Sudden onset; mixing past and present; disorientation; poor short-term memory; easily startled; paranoia.

Yes ↓

**Is it terminal agitation?** —Yes→ Sedate promptly (with midazolam and/or methotrimeprazine). Re-assess once the patient is settled.

No ↓

**Is the patient liable to harm themselves or others?** —Yes→ **Is it possible to manage the patient without sedation if familiar carers are present?** —No→ Sedate (eg haloperidol) 10 mg

Yes ↘ Support the carers

No ↓

**Is the patient frightened?** —Yes→

No ↓

**Have I talked to the relatives to search for clues as to the cause?** —No→ <u>Ask about:</u>
– sudden onset?
– head trauma (subdural)?
– alcohol intake?
– recent drug change?
– insulin excess?

Yes ↓

**Have I examined the patient and `screened' for reversible causes?** —No→ Confusion is worsened by uncontrolled pain. Examine bladder and rectum. See note.

Yes ↓

**Is the patient's environment as calm and stable as possible?** —No→ **KEY PART of managing the situation.** Confusion often gradually settles when the patient's environment is calm and stable.

Yes ↓

**Have I given enough explanation to relatives <u>AND</u> patient?** —No→ **KEY PART of managing the situation.** Relatives are frightened and the patient often has partial insight or lucid intervals.

↓

Monitor mental state and reduce sedation when possible

10

## Is it confusion or dementia?

Confusion can be reversible but dementia is not. Confusion is usually of sudden onset, over days and dementia is of gradual onset, over months. Confusion is usually obvious (rambling speech, poor memory for recent events, disorientation, drowsy yet easily startled) but remember that the patient may have both dementia and confusion, or neither – they may just be deaf, grumpy and out of their normal environment.

## Is it terminal agitation?

If the patient is dying, confused and agitated (physical and mentally) it is usually best (for both the patient and the relatives) to sedate promptly (with midazolam and\or methotrimeprazine), then re-assess the situation and consider reducing sedation. High doses may be needed. Is there a reversible reason (eg urinary retention).

## Is it alcohol withdrawal?

Sudden severe agitation suggests 'delirium tremens' due to alcohol withdrawal in an alcoholic. The best solution in advanced illness is often to restore a reasonable alcohol intake.

## Is there a reversible cause?

Ask relatives about recent drug changes, examine carefully (especially bladder and rectum) and check blood glucose, calcium, urea electrolytes. Send a MSU to exclude UTI.

## Is a CT scan indicated?

Consider a CT scan if there has been a head injury within recent weeks, (a subdural haematoma may be treatable) or if there are neurological signs suggestive of brain metastases

## Is the patient lucid at times?

Lucid intervals often occur (usually in the morning) when it is possible to converse with the patient, and discover their wishes about management options.

## Is the environment calm?

The most important part of management is to create a calm stable environment (quiet, dim lighting, familiar faces). A familiar relative to sit with the patient can be very calming (but the relative may need a lot of support). The patient may need admitting from home. Confusion is the most difficult symptom to manage at home, because it tends to erode the carer's emotional energy for coping – consider admission.

## Is sedation needed?

Confusion may not be distressing (and we then tend to say the patient is "pleasantly confused") but it may be very frightening. Acknowledging the patient's fear can help to calm the patient.

## Are the relatives getting enough support?

Confusion is frightening for the relatives. Explanation helps (likely cause, likely course of events etc).

# CONSTIPATION

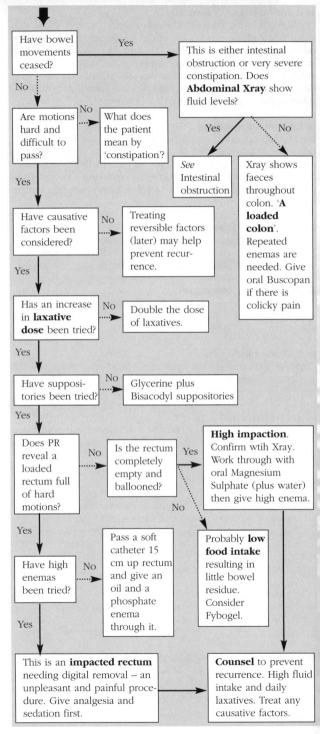

Have bowel movements ceased? — **Yes** → This is either intestinal obstruction or very severe constipation. Does **Abdominal Xray** show fluid levels?

**No** ⋯→ Are motions hard and difficult to pass? — **No** ⋯→ What does the patient mean by 'constipation'?

Does **Abdominal Xray** show fluid levels? — **Yes** → *See* Intestinal obstruction

**No** ⋯→ Xray shows faeces throughout colon. '**A loaded colon**'. Repeated enemas are needed. Give oral Buscopan if there is colicky pain

Are motions hard and difficult to pass? **Yes** ↓

Have causative factors been considered? — **No** ⋯→ Treating reversible factors (later) may help prevent recurrence.

**Yes** ↓

Has an increase in **laxative dose** been tried? — **No** ⋯→ Double the dose of laxatives.

**Yes** ↓

Have suppositories been tried? — **No** ⋯→ Glycerine plus Bisacodyl suppositories

**Yes** ↓

Does PR reveal a loaded rectum full of hard motions? — **No** ⋯→ Is the rectum completely empty and ballooned? — **Yes** → **High impaction**. Confirm with Xray. Work through with oral Magnesium Sulphate (plus water) then give high enema.

Is the rectum completely empty and ballooned? **No** ⋯→ Probably **low food intake** resulting in little bowel residue. Consider Fybogel.

**Yes** ↓

Have high enemas been tried? — **No** ⋯→ Pass a soft catheter 15 cm up rectum and give an oil and a phosphate enema through it.

**Yes** ↓

This is an **impacted rectum** needing digital removal – an unpleasant and painful procedure. Give analgesia and sedation first.

**Counsel** to prevent recurrence. High fluid intake and daily laxatives. Treat any causative factors.

## Is the patient constipated?

Some patients use "constipation" to mean less frequent bowel movement, but constipation means difficulty passing motions – usually because they are hard. It is a common problem and can be extremely distressing. One patient wrote in her diary – "Analgesics freeze your pain, but they freeze up your bowels as well".

## Is it causing other symptoms?

Severe constipation can cause colicky pain in the abdomen (which can radiate to the groin, chest and back) anorexia, malaise, nausea and vomiting and in the elderly confusion.

## Is it causing "diarrhoea"?

Severe constipation can present as spurious diarrhoea, with small amounts of liquid faeces passing around the sides of a rectal bolus, often with some faecal incontinence.

## Are faeces impacted?

It is important to do a rectal examination whenever it is suspected ("if you don't put your finger in you put your foot in"). In high constipation the rectum can be empty and ballooned. If there is doubt about the diagnosis a plain abdominal Xray will show faeces throughout the colon. For disimpaction give IM diamorphine 2.5mg (or more if on regular morphine) with midazolam 5–10mg, prior to the procedure.

## How can it be prevented?

The best policy is aggressive prevention. Prescribe DAILY laxatives and start the same day morphine is started (eg Co-danthramer 20 ml nocte). The main aim of laxative use is an easy bowel action, not necessarily a daily one. Nevertheless it is a good idea to teach the patient the "3-day rule" – If the bowels are not open after 3 days a micro-enema or suppositories are needed (eg 5mg bisacodyl plus one glycerine suppository – which normally work within an hour).

## Is there a contributory cause?

Common contributing factors (in addition to morphine) include dehydration, drugs (anti-cholinergics, vincristine, ondansetron) and difficulty getting access to a toilet or commode. Consider changing morphine to fentanyl patch.

# DEHYDRATION

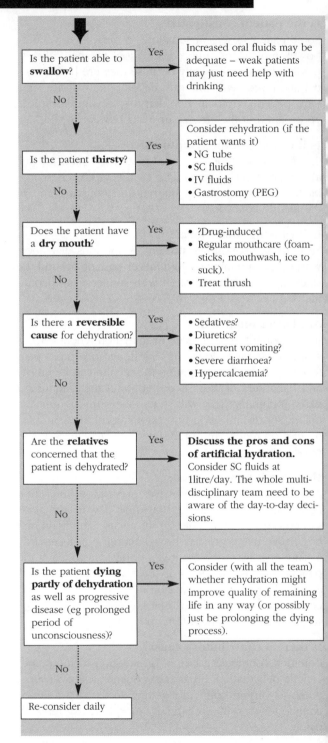

Is the patient able to **swallow**?

Yes → Increased oral fluids may be adequate – weak patients may just need help with drinking

No ↓

Is the patient **thirsty**?

Yes → Consider rehydration (if the patient wants it)
- NG tube
- SC fluids
- IV fluids
- Gastrostomy (PEG)

No ↓

Does the patient have a **dry mouth**?

Yes → 
- ?Drug-induced
- Regular mouthcare (foam-sticks, mouthwash, ice to suck).
- Treat thrush

No ↓

Is there a **reversible cause** for dehydration?

Yes → 
- Sedatives?
- Diuretics?
- Recurrent vomiting?
- Severe diarrhoea?
- Hypercalcaemia?

No ↓

Are the **relatives** concerned that the patient is dehydrated?

Yes → **Discuss the pros and cons of artificial hydration.** Consider SC fluids at 1litre/day. The whole multi-disciplinary team need to be aware of the day-to-day decisions.

No ↓

Is the patient **dying partly of dehydration** as well as progressive disease (eg prolonged period of unconsciousness)?

Yes → Consider (with all the team) whether rehydration might improve quality of remaining life in any way (or possibly just be prolonging the dying process).

No ↓

Re-consider daily

**Is the patient dehydrated?**

Dry tongue, sunken eyes, inelastic skin, fast pulse, poor urine output (and dark urine) all suggest dehydration. Sodium urea and albumin levels may be elevated. The patient may not be thirsty.

**Is re-hydration indicated?**

Towards death, a person's desire for food and drink lessens. Artificial hydration does not normally improve comfort or survival. IV re-hydration is usually indicated if there is a possibility of a potentially correctable cause (eg excessive diuretics, sedation, recurrent vomiting, diarrhoea or hypercalcaemia).

**Is a dry mouth the main problem?**

Some dehydration commonly occurs when a dying patient becomes too weak to swallow. Dry mouth is common but responds to good mouth care (reassess any medication that may be contributing to it). Artificial hydration is unnecessary just for dry mouth.

**Is the patient thirsty?**

If the patient is thirsty they should be re-hydrated, orally if possible. Hydration of semi-conscious patients in the hospice or nursing home setting is easier to achieve now that the subcutaneous route has become commonly used for fluid, (eg 1 litre of normal saline or 5% glucose per 12-24 hours by SC infusion – usually in the thigh or abdomen). 3l per day can be infused if necessary by using 2 sites. 1500 units of hyaluronidase (Hyalase) is sometimes used to prime the line to help the fluid diffuse into the subcutaneous tissues – but it is not essential.

**Should a hospice have a policy about re-hydration?**

No. The appropriateness of artificial hydration continues to depend on regular assessment of the likely benefits and burdens of such intervention. A blanket policy of either always giving artificial hydration, or of no artificial hydration, is ethically indefensible. The appropriateness of artificial hydration for a patient should be judged on a day-to-day basis, weighing up the potential harms and benefits. The decisions should involve the multi-professional team, the patient, and relatives and carers, but the senior doctor has ultimate responsibility for the decision. A competent patient has the right to refuse artificial hydration, even if it is considered of clinical benefit. Incompetent patients retain this right through a valid advance refusal.

*See also*: Terminal phase

# DIARRHOEA

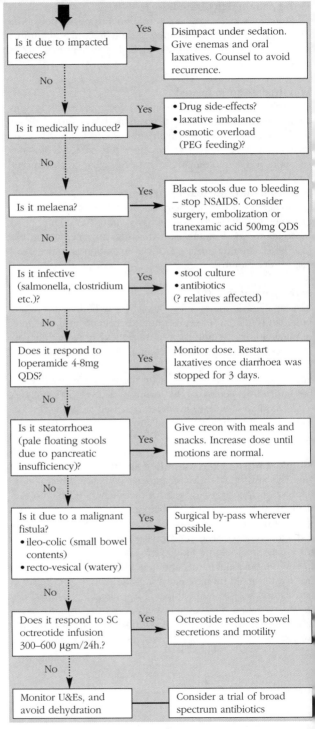

Is it due to impacted faeces? — **Yes** → Disimpact under sedation. Give enemas and oral laxatives. Counsel to avoid recurrence.

**No** ↓

Is it medically induced? — **Yes** →
- Drug side-effects?
- laxative imbalance
- osmotic overload (PEG feeding)?

**No** ↓

Is it melaena? — **Yes** → Black stools due to bleeding – stop NSAIDS. Consider surgery, embolization or tranexamic acid 500mg QDS

**No** ↓

Is it infective (salmonella, clostridium etc.)? — **Yes** →
- stool culture
- antibiotics
(? relatives affected)

**No** ↓

Does it respond to loperamide 4-8mg QDS? — **Yes** → Monitor dose. Restart laxatives once diarrhoea was stopped for 3 days.

**No** ↓

Is it steatorrhoea (pale floating stools due to pancreatic insufficiency)? — **Yes** → Give creon with meals and snacks. Increase dose until motions are normal.

**No** ↓

Is it due to a malignant fistula?
- ileo-colic (small bowel contents)
- recto-vesical (watery)
— **Yes** → Surgical by-pass wherever possible.

**No** ↓

Does it respond to SC octreotide infusion 300–600 μgm/24h.? — **Yes** → Octreotide reduces bowel secretions and motility

**No** ↓

Monitor U&Es, and avoid dehydration — Consider a trial of broad spectrum antibiotics

## Is it due to impacted faeces?

This is the commonest cause of diarrhoea in the hospice setting. Small amounts of liquid motion (sometimes with incontinence) suggest overflow past an impacted lump of faeces in the rectum. There is a history of severe constipation before the diarrhoea started. Digital evacuation is needed, then education about the use of laxatives.

## Is it due to excess laxatives?

Patients commonly get into a cycle of laxative misuse (getting a bit constipated, taking too much laxative, having diarrhoea, stopping the laxatives, getting constipated). Teach regular daily use of laxatives. Diarrhoea may be also a side-effect of other drugs (eg antibiotics).

## Is it melaena?

Black tarry stools suggests bleeding higher up the bowel. Test for blood and check the Hb level. Blood transfusion is only indicated if the bleeding can be controlled.<None>

## Is it infective?

Sudden onset of diarrhoea and vomiting together strongly suggests gastro-enteritis is the cause. Have others been affected? Send stool cultures and take advice from the bacteriologist about treatment.

## Is it malabsorbtion?

Cancer of the pancreas (and sometimes other upper abdominal malignancies) can cause obstruction to the pancreatic duct and malabsorbtion of fat causing frequent smelly pale motions that tend to float. Loperamide is ineffective but it responds well to pancreatic enzyme therapy such as creon (1–3 with meals and 1 with snacks or milky drinks).

## Is it due to a fistula?

Persistent diarrhoea in a patient with intra-abdominal malignancy suggests a fistula may have occurred. A fistula from the small bowel into the colon causes undigested small bowel contents to pass very rapidly through the bowel. If surgical repair is not an option treat with octreotide.

## Is it severe enough to cause dehydration?

Check U&Es and consider rehydration. Chronic diarrhoea can cause low potassium levels.

# DYSPHAGIA

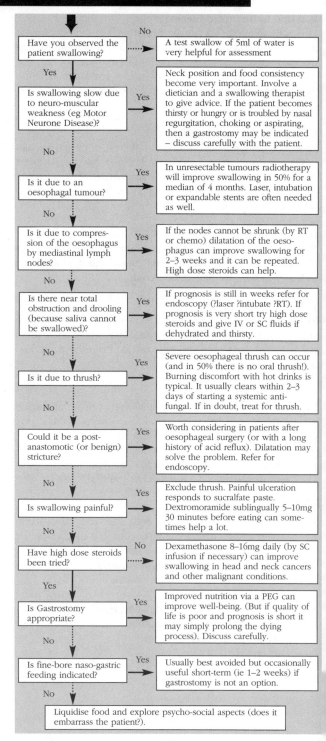

Have you observed the patient swallowing? → No → A test swallow of 5ml of water is very helpful for assessment

Yes ↓

Is swallowing slow due to neuro-muscular weakness (eg Motor Neurone Disease)? → Yes → Neck position and food consistency become very important. Involve a dietician and a swallowing therapist to give advice. If the patient becomes thirsty or hungry or is troubled by nasal regurgitation, choking or aspirating, then a gastrostomy may be indicated – discuss carefully with the patient.

No ↓

Is it due to an oesophagal tumour? → Yes → In unresectable tumours radiotherapy will improve swallowing in 50% for a median of 4 months. Laser, intubation or expandable stents are often needed as well.

No ↓

Is it due to compression of the oesophagus by mediastinal lymph nodes? → Yes → If the nodes cannot be shrunk (by RT or chemo) dilatation of the oesophagus can improve swallowing for 2–3 weeks and it can be repeated. High dose steroids can help.

No ↓

Is there near total obstruction and drooling (because saliva cannot be swallowed)? → Yes → If prognosis is still in weeks refer for endoscopy (?laser ?intubate ?RT). If prognosis is very short try high dose steroids and give IV or SC fluids if dehydrated and thirsty.

No ↓

Is it due to thrush? → Yes → Severe oesophageal thrush can occur (and in 50% there is no oral thrush!). Burning discomfort with hot drinks is typical. It usually clears within 2–3 days of starting a systemic anti-fungal. If in doubt, treat for thrush.

No ↓

Could it be a post-anastomotic (or benign) stricture? → Yes → Worth considering in patients after oesophageal surgery (or with a long history of acid reflux). Dilatation may solve the problem. Refer for endoscopy.

No ↓

Is swallowing painful? → Yes → Exclude thrush. Painful ulceration responds to sucralfate paste. Dextromoramide sublingually 5–10mg 30 minutes before eating can sometimes help a lot.

No ↓

Have high dose steroids been tried? → No → Dexamethasone 8–16mg daily (by SC infusion if necessary) can improve swallowing in head and neck cancers and other malignant conditions.

Yes ↓

Is Gastrostomy appropriate? → Yes → Improved nutrition via a PEG can improve well-being. (But if quality of life is poor and prognosis is short it may simply prolong the dying process). Discuss carefully.

No ↓

Is fine-bore naso-gastric feeding indicated? → Yes → Usually best avoided but occasionally useful short-term (ie 1–2 weeks) if gastrostomy is not an option.

No ↓

Liquidise food and explore psycho-social aspects (does it embarrass the patient?).

**What is the main problem?**
Is the problem reduced hydration, reduced nutrition, loss of social pleasure, pain on swallowing or risk of aspiration?. Are the relatives distressed by the poor food intake?

**What is the cause?**
Patients localise the level accurately in 99% of cases. Observe a TEST SWALLOW of 5ml of water to visualize the problem. Is it a problem with saliva, chewing (dentures or teeth), oral cavity (mucosal pain, poor closure) tongue movement ("ta" tests anterior tongue, "ka" tests posterior tongue) elevation of palate (nasal regurgitation) or closure of epiglottis (coughing, choking) elevation of larynx or oesophageal peristalsis?. Note that the gag reflex is irrelevant to the swallowing reflex.

**Is it a delayed pharyngeal phase?**
Pharyngeal function can be assessed at the bedside. Laryngeal elevation is easy to feel and normally takes 1 second. If it takes 5 seconds or longer swallowing becomes hard work and there is a risk of inadequate intake. Changing neck and body position (and food consistency) can still improve swallowing – involve a swallowing therapist and dietician. If it takes longer than 10 seconds then non-oral feeding will usually be needed. Is it worsened by drugs (eg metoclopramide)?

**Is aspiration occurring?**
After a test swallow ask the patient to say "Ahh". A gurgling noise means aspiration is probably occurring. Aspiration is symptomless in 40% of cases. In 60% it causes choking, coughing, drooling or recurrent chest infections. Consider changing the neck position (holding neck forward reduces it) and food changing consistency may help (eg semi-solids like yoghurt and custard can reduce aspiration occurring). If severe, non-oral feeding is necessary. Barium swallow is unhelpful (and can be dangerous). Video fluoroscopy will demonstrate the cause of problem and show how much aspiration is occurring.

**Is non-oral feeding needed?**
   – fine-bore NG tube (1-2 week only)
   – PEG
   – open gastrostomy (eg oesophageal block)
   – pharyngostomy (for oral tumours)

Improved nutrition can help well-being (and relieve nutritional deficiencies) and should be considered early in patients with a reasonable prognosis. Seek advice of specialist nutritional nurse. (Note that it is easier to start non-oral feeding than to stop.)

**Is the patient in the last few days?**
The key decision is: "Is the patient thirsty?" If not, focus on mouth care. (see Dehydration).

# DYSPNOEA

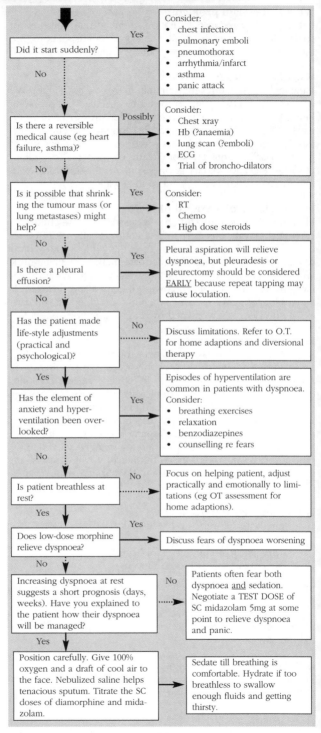

**Did it start suddenly?** — Yes →
Consider:
- chest infection
- pulmonary emboli
- pneumothorax
- arrhythmia/infarct
- asthma
- panic attack

No ↓

**Is there a reversible medical cause (eg heart failure, asthma)?** — Possibly →
Consider:
- Chest xray
- Hb (?anaemia)
- lung scan (?emboli)
- ECG
- Trial of broncho-dilators

No ↓

**Is it possible that shrinking the tumour mass (or lung metastases) might help?** — Yes →
Consider:
- RT
- Chemo
- High dose steroids

No ↓

**Is there a pleural effusion?** — Yes →
Pleural aspiration will relieve dyspnoea, but pleuradesis or pleurectomy should be considered <u>EARLY</u> because repeat tapping may cause loculation.

No ↓

**Has the patient made life-style adjustments (practical and psychological)?** — No →
Discuss limitations. Refer to O.T. for home adaptions and diversional therapy

Yes ↓

**Has the element of anxiety and hyper-ventilation been over-looked?** — Yes →
Episodes of hyperventilation are common in patients with dyspnoea. Consider:
- breathing exercises
- relaxation
- benzodiazepines
- counselling re fears

No ↓

**Is patient breathless at rest?** — No →
Focus on helping patient, adjust practically and emotionally to limitations (eg OT assessment for home adaptions).

Yes ↓

**Does low-dose morphine relieve dyspnoea?** — Yes →
Discuss fears of dyspnoea worsening

No ↓

**Increasing dyspnoea at rest suggests a short prognosis (days, weeks). Have you explained to the patient how their dyspnoea will be managed?** — No →
Patients often fear both dyspnoea <u>and</u> sedation. Negotiate a TEST DOSE of SC midazolam 5mg at some point to relieve dyspnoea and panic.

Yes ↓

Position carefully. Give 100% oxygen and a draft of cool air to the face. Nebulized saline helps tenacious sputum. Titrate the SC doses of diamorphine and mida-zolam.

Sedate till breathing is comfortable. Hydrate if too breathless to swallow enough fluids and getting thirsty.

**Did the dyspnoea (breathlessness) start suddenly?**
Sudden onset over hours suggests a medical cause (myocardial infarct, embolus, arrythmia, asthma). These may need excluding before diagnosing a first panic attack. Consider a CXR and ECG. Worsening over days suggests a chest infection or pleural effusion. Worsening over weeks suggests anaemia or tumour progression.

**Is it mainly on exertion?**
Breathlessness on exertion is the commonest problem (which may gradually worsen). The focus of management is on non-drug measures. The patient has to learn to *avoid* distressing breathlessness by adjusting their life-style (a home visit by an occupational therapist can be very helpful) and has to learn to *cope* with the sensation when it occurs without panicking (breathing exercises and relaxation techniques taught by a physiotherapist can be very effective).

**What does it prevent the patient from doing?**
This is a useful question to assess the impact on quality of life. Most patients have difficulty coping with some aspects of change in life-style, and need help adjusting (practical and emotional).

**Should breathless patients still take exercise?**
Suprisingly breathless patients should still exercise to the limits of comfort, because exercise has a positive effect physically and mentally. Relatives are often over-protective and try to stop the patient from doing anything. An assessment of exercise tolerance by the doctor, using a simple walking test, can give the patient and relatives more confidence.

**Is the patient breathless at rest?**
Difficulty breathing even at rest (or taking a long time to recover from exertion) is when low dose morphine is considered (a starting dose is 2.5mg morphine 4 hourly) and it can greatly reduce the distressing sensation of breathlessness.

**Is the patient getting episodes of hyperventilation?**
Breathlessness is frightening and many patients with breathlessness *also* get episodes of hyperventilation, and sometimes panic. A helpful point is that breathing tends to ease slightly with exertion if hyperventilation is the main problem. Ask if the patient feels frightened at times. Most patients fear it will worsen and they will die gasping for breath. Open discussion of fears (usually about it worsening) and how it can be controlled (if it worsens) can help a lot.

**How is severe breathlessness at rest managed?**
This can occur in the last few days of life, and breathing can become more and more distressing. SC infusion of diamorphine plus midazolam in carefully titrated doses is effective. Continuous oxygen is also helpful (but constant fears about the oxygen cylinders running out is not, so change them regularly). Skilled nursing, and careful positioning and moving of the patient make all the difference. Make sure the environment feels safe and calm and that the patient is not left alone. Patients often fear it getting worse, but also fear sedation in case they stop breathing altogether. Negotiate the idea of a TEST DOSE OF MIDAZOLAM 5mg IM with the patient. This gives sedation and relief without depressing respiration, and wears off after an hour or so. If the patient is too breathless to speak arrange a signal so they can ask to try it when they feel ready, which gives them an important sense of control.

# FENTANYL 1 – USAGE

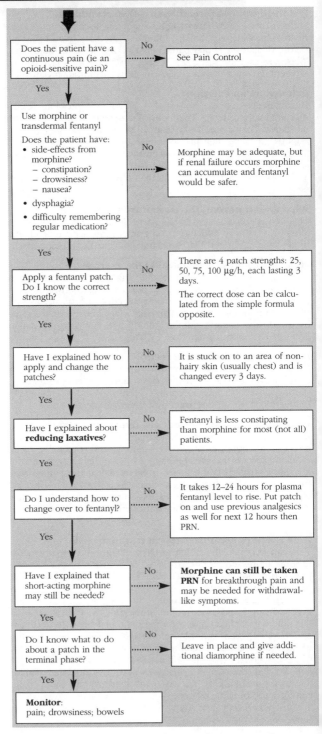

Does the patient have a continuous pain (ie an opioid-sensitive pain)?
→ No → See Pain Control

↓ Yes

Use morphine or transdermal fentanyl

Does the patient have:
- side-effects from morphine?
  - constipation?
  - drowsiness?
  - nausea?
- dysphagia?
- difficulty remembering regular medication?

→ No → Morphine may be adequate, but if renal failure occurs morphine can accumulate and fentanyl would be safer.

↓ Yes

Apply a fentanyl patch. Do I know the correct strength?
→ No → There are 4 patch strengths: 25, 50, 75, 100 µg/h, each lasting 3 days.

The correct dose can be calculated from the simple formula opposite.

↓ Yes

Have I explained how to apply and change the patches?
→ No → It is stuck on to an area of non-hairy skin (usually chest) and is changed every 3 days.

↓ Yes

Have I explained about **reducing laxatives**?
→ No → Fentanyl is less constipating than morphine for most (not all) patients.

↓ Yes

Do I understand how to change over to fentanyl?
→ No → It takes 12–24 hours for plasma fentanyl level to rise. Put patch on and use previous analgesics as well for next 12 hours then PRN.

↓ Yes

Have I explained that short-acting morphine may still be needed?
→ No → **Morphine can still be taken PRN** for breakthrough pain and may be needed for withdrawal-like symptoms.

↓ Yes

Do I know what to do about a patch in the terminal phase?
→ No → Leave in place and give additional diamorphine if needed.

↓ Yes

**Monitor:**
pain; drowsiness; bowels

## Which patch strength is needed?

1. It is safe to start the 25mcg per hour patch if the patient has a constant pain which has not responded to moderate analgesics such as 60mg of Codeine 4 hourly or 2 Co-proxamol tablets 4 hourly. If the patient is already taking morphine and is being converted to a Fentanyl patch the correct patch strength can be calculated from the simple formula below.

| 4 hourly **oral morphine** (mg) (× 6 for 24h dose) | **Fentanyl patch** (mcg\hr) |
|:---:|:---:|
| 5–20mg | 25 |
| 30mg | 50 |
| 45mg | 75 |
| 60mg | 100 |
| 120mg | 200 |

## When can the patch be started?

Apply the first patch at night together with the usual night dose of morphine then phase out the regular morphine dose the following day. The patient can still use immediate release morphine PRN for any breakthrough pain.

## What are the side-effects?

Constipation, nausea or drowsiness can occur but there is a lower incidence than with morphine. Prolonged fever or a hot bath can increase fentanyl release and the chance of side-effects. Side-effects may persist for 24 hours after the patch is removed.

## Is there a maximum dose?

There is no maximum dose of fentanyl but if the dose required exceeds 300mcg per hour (ie three 100 µg/h patches) consider additional or alternative analgesic therapy.

## Is it a controlled drug?

Fentanyl is a controlled drug therefore prescriptions need to be written by the prescribing doctor in figures and words eg "Durogesic 25mgm per hour × 5 (five) patches, apply 1 patch every 3 days."

## Can Fentanyl be used in the terminal phase?

Fentanyl should not be prescribed for the first time if the patient is in the terminal phase (ie their condition is deteriorating day by day) because it can be difficult to find the right dose quickly in a changing situation. However if the patient already has a Fentanyl patch this can be left in place and oral morphine or IM diamorphine can be given for breakthrough pain. A safe starting dose of IM diamorphine is 5mg per 25mcg per hour of Fentanyl.

## What is the chance of a morphine withdrawal reaction?

About 10% of patients may experience transient withdrawal like symptoms when converted from morphine to fentanyl. The symptoms can last from a few days to 2 weeks and include diarrhoea, flu-like symptoms, yawning, runny nose, colic, anxiety, shivering and occasionally hallucinations. These symptoms respond within 30-60 minutes to a small dose of immediate release morphine eg Sevredol 10mg which can be given as often as necessary until it settles down.

*See also*: Fentanyl 2 – about the patch

## <u>Durogesic – The Fentanyl Patch</u>

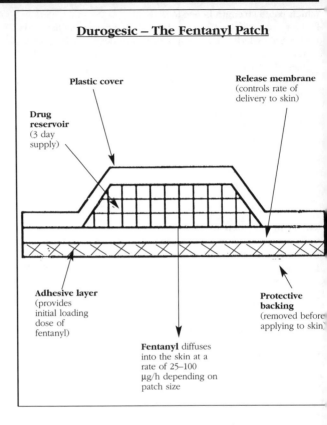

**Plastic cover**

**Release membrane**
(controls rate of
delivery to skin)

**Drug
reservoir**
(3 day
supply)

**Adhesive layer**
(provides
initial loading
dose of
fentanyl)

**Protective
backing**
(removed before
applying to skin)

**Fentanyl** diffuses
into the skin at a
rate of 25–100
μg/h depending on
patch size

There are 4 patch strengths:

25 μg/hour
50 μg/hour
75 μg/hour
100 μg/hour

# FENTANYL 2 – ABOUT THE PATCH

## Where is the patch stuck on?

The patch is stuck on flat skin on the upper body (front or back) or upper arm. The skin should not have any cuts or spots and should not be hairy. Hairs can be cut with a pair of scissors but skin should not be shaved, as this may affect absorption. The skin should be dry. Soaps, oils or lotions should be avoided. The patch should be pressed firmly in place for 30 seconds and the edges of the patch pressed down.

## How often is it changed?

The patch is normally changed every 3rd day (eg if it is put on at 9am on Wednesday it should be exchanged for a new patch at 9am of Saturday). Several days should elapse before a new patch is applied to the same area of skin.

Occasionally some patients notice that the analgesic effect falls after 60 hours, and it may then be necessary to change the patch every 2 days.

## Can allergy to the patch occur?

Allergy is rare. Most skin reactions (redness or itching) resolve within 24 hours of removal of the patch. Occasionally they are troublesome and an alternative form of analgesia has to be found.

## What if the patch falls off?

If a patch falls off it is safe to apply another replacement patch straight away and this new replacement patch will last a further 3 days. If the patch begins to peel off use Micropore or Tegaderm to hold it in place.

## Is it waterproof?

The patch is waterproof for a shower, bath or swimming. The patch should not be worn under a tight elasticated band. Direct heat should be avoided as it can increase the rate of release of fentanyl (eg heat pads, hot water bottles, electric blankets, heat lamps, saunas, spa baths). Tell the patient to cover the patch with clothing if they sunbathe or use a sunbed.

## What about used patches?

Used patches should be folded in half so that the sticky side sticks to itself and should be put back into its original pouch (which should therefore be kept when the patch is first opened). It is safe to discard the pouch in the household rubbish but keep out of the reach of children or pets.

# LYMPHOEDEMA

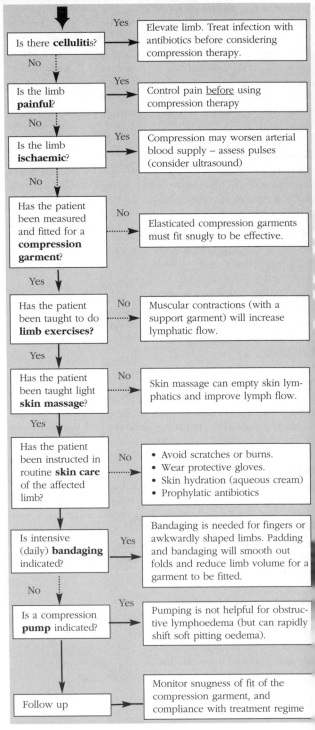

**Is there cellulitis?** — Yes → Elevate limb. Treat infection with antibiotics before considering compression therapy.

No

**Is the limb painful?** — Yes → Control pain before using compression therapy

No

**Is the limb ischaemic?** — Yes → Compression may worsen arterial blood supply – assess pulses (consider ultrasound)

No

**Has the patient been measured and fitted for a compression garment?** — No → Elasticated compression garments must fit snugly to be effective.

Yes

**Has the patient been taught to do limb exercises?** — No → Muscular contractions (with a support garment) will increase lymphatic flow.

Yes

**Has the patient been taught light skin massage?** — No → Skin massage can empty skin lymphatics and improve lymph flow.

Yes

**Has the patient been instructed in routine skin care of the affected limb?** — No →
- Avoid scratches or burns.
- Wear protective gloves.
- Skin hydration (aqueous cream)
- Prophylatic antibiotics

**Is intensive (daily) bandaging indicated?** — Yes → Bandaging is needed for fingers or awkwardly shaped limbs. Padding and bandaging will smooth out folds and reduce limb volume for a garment to be fitted.

No

**Is a compression pump indicated?** — Yes → Pumping is not helpful for obstructive lymphoedema (but can rapidly shift soft pitting oedema).

**Follow up** → Monitor snugness of fit of the compression garment, and compliance with treatment regime

## What is lymphoedema?

Lymphoedema means the swelling of the limb due to lymphatic obstruction. It causes a heavy and uncomfortable arm or leg, restricts movement and eventually causes skin thickening. An important part of management is teaching the patient and carer about control of the swelling. It can be hard for patients to realise that there is no cure and the management regime is "for life".

## Is it a recent problem?

Recent onset lymphoedema is usually easier to shift. It is occasionally reversible (for a time) with high dose steroids.

## Is there truncal oedema?

Oedema of the chest wall or abdomen can only be shifted by massage, and suggests a more severe problem.

## How can massage help?

Stimulates lymph flow in the superficial lymph vessels which stimulates the normal lymphatic contractions and can milk lymph away from swollen area (massage starts in the <u>healthy</u> area and works towards the affected area). It must be demonstrated and taught properly.

## Does the compression garment fit properly?

It is essential the support fits snugly. The patient's limb needs to be measured first. Good compression garments are made by Medi. Awkwardly-shaped limbs may need a special made-to-measure sleeve (eg Biersdorf).

## Should exercises be recommended?

Limb exercise increases lymphatic flow, especially when using a compression garment and are an important part of management. Passive limb movements help if the patient is too weak to exercise.

## Is bandaging necessary?

Bandaging with low pressure elastic bandages (eg secure 40) is useful for awkwardly-shaped limbs, finger swelling or lymphorrhoea.

## Should a compression pump be used?

Compression pumps are not used routinely. They can be of benefit to rapidly clear soft oedema. They should be used at low pressure. They should not be used if there is trunk swelling. Sequential (multi-chamber) pumps are more effective than single chamber pumps.

## Should diuretics be prescribed?

Diuretics are usually ineffective unless there is an element of venous obstruction and some pitting oedema superimposed on lymphoedema.

## Is recurrent cellulitis a problem?

Damaged lymphatics are susceptible to infection, (which then cause further damage). Infection can be blood-born (ie can occur even without skin damage). Teach skin care and give prophylactic antibiotics.

# MORPHINE

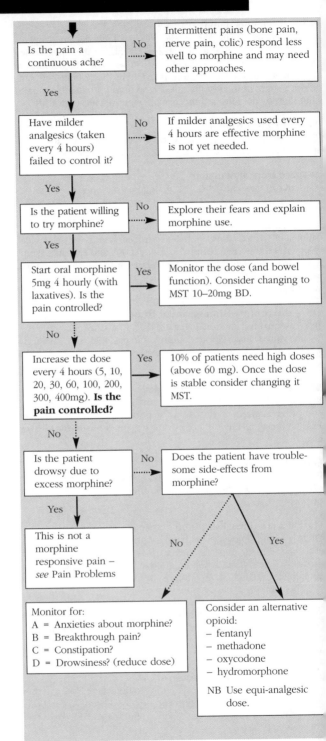

Is the pain a continuous ache? — **No** ····▶ Intermittent pains (bone pain, nerve pain, colic) respond less well to morphine and may need other approaches.

**Yes** ↓

Have milder analgesics (taken every 4 hours) failed to control it? — **No** ····▶ If milder analgesics used every 4 hours are effective morphine is not yet needed.

**Yes** ↓

Is the patient willing to try morphine? — **No** ····▶ Explore their fears and explain morphine use.

**Yes** ↓

Start oral morphine 5mg 4 hourly (with laxatives). Is the pain controlled? — **Yes** ➔ Monitor the dose (and bowel function). Consider changing to MST 10–20mg BD.

**No** ↓

Increase the dose every 4 hours (5, 10, 20, 30, 60, 100, 200, 300, 400mg). **Is the pain controlled?** — **Yes** ➔ 10% of patients need high doses (above 60 mg). Once the dose is stable consider changing it MST.

**No** ↓

Is the patient drowsy due to excess morphine? — **No** ····▶ Does the patient have troublesome side-effects from morphine?

**Yes** ↓

This is not a morphine responsive pain – *see* Pain Problems

No ↙          Yes ↘

Monitor for:
A = Anxieties about morphine?
B = Breakthrough pain?
C = Constipation?
D = Drowsiness? (reduce dose)

Consider an alternative opioid:
– fentanyl
– methadone
– oxycodone
– hydromorphone

NB Use equi-analgesic dose.

**When should morphine be started?**

Morphine should be considered for any continuous pain that has not responded to other analgesics. Take a careful analgesic history before prescribing morphine – the doses of the analgesics used guide you about whether morphine is needed and also the correct starting dose, usually 5-10 mg 4 hourly, or 2.5 mg in the elderly or frail, or if it is for dyspnoea rather than for pain.

**Is the patient frightened of using morphine?**

Many patients (and families) fear that if you have cancer and morphine is prescribed it means "the beginning of the end" or the fear may be of addiction or of "becoming a zombie". Ask directly "Do you have any particular worries about taking morphine?" Explain that when used for pain (ie opioid-responsive pain) there is no danger of addiction, and even if taken for some time, stopping it may cause the pain to recur but will not cause "cold turkey" symptoms of goose-bumps, shivering, agitation etc. Similarly there is no danger of "becoming a zombie" if the dose is balanced carefully.

**Does the patient understand the principles of balancing the dose?**

It is important to spend some time explaining how the dose is monitored. If the pain persists then the regular dose is increased (but remains 4 hourly) but if the pain is controlled and the patient feels drowsy then the dose is reduced. Every day the patient needs to ask: "do I still have pain, am I feeling drowsy".

**How often should the dose be changed?**

On the first day the dose may need to be adjusted every 4 hours if the pain is not coming under control. For the next few days, it may only be necessary to adjust the dose every 24 hours or so. Once the dose is steady change over to a modified release morphine, with some immediate-release morphine for PRN use.

**Is there fear about increasing the dose?**

Some patients fear the dose going up "in case it no longer works when the pain gets very severe" or in case it means the disease is worsening and the end is nearing. Explain that there is no maximum dose, that the aim is to keep the patient free of pain, that there are no medals for suffering pain, that pain does not co-relate with disease progression and most importantly explain that the dose needed by each person is very individual, and needing a high dose may partly be due to a more efficient metabolism of morphine.

**When should laxatives be started?**

Almost every patient on morphine will get constipated (unless they already have a tendency to diarrhoea). Start laxatives on day 1, eg co-danthramer capsules 1-2 each night, and explain the "3 day rule": a suppository if no bowel movement for 3 days, and increase the daily laxative dose. The laxative dose may need to be increased if the morphine dose is increased.

**How often should a patient on morphine be monitored?**

Once the dose is steady and the patient is confident about how to use morphine, it is only necessary to see the patient every few weeks, telling them to ask for immediate advice if the pain control is lost.

# NAUSEA AND VOMITING

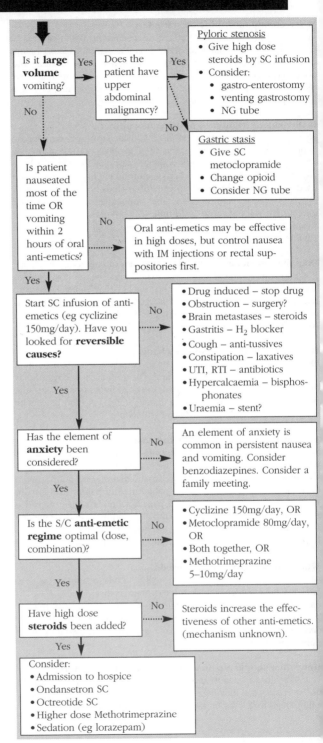

**Is it large volume vomiting?** — Yes → **Does the patient have upper abdominal malignancy?** — Yes →

Pyloric stenosis
- Give high dose steroids by SC infusion
- Consider:
  - gastro-enterostomy
  - venting gastrostomy
  - NG tube

No ↓

**Does the patient have upper abdominal malignancy?** — No →

Gastric stasis
- Give SC metoclopramide
- Change opioid
- Consider NG tube

No ↓

**Is patient nauseated most of the time OR vomiting within 2 hours of oral anti-emetics?** — No →

Oral anti-emetics may be effective in high doses, but control nausea with IM injections or rectal suppositories first.

Yes ↓

**Start SC infusion of anti-emetics (eg cyclizine 150mg/day). Have you looked for reversible causes?** — No →

- Drug induced – stop drug
- Obstruction – surgery?
- Brain metastases – steroids
- Gastritis – $H_2$ blocker
- Cough – anti-tussives
- Constipation – laxatives
- UTI, RTI – antibiotics
- Hypercalcaemia – bisphosphonates
- Uraemia – stent?

Yes ↓

**Has the element of anxiety been considered?** — No →

An element of anxiety is common in persistent nausea and vomiting. Consider benzodiazepines. Consider a family meeting.

Yes ↓

**Is the S/C anti-emetic regime optimal (dose, combination)?** — No →

- Cyclizine 150mg/day, OR
- Metoclopramide 80mg/day, OR
- Both together, OR
- Methotrimeprazine 5–10mg/day

Yes ↓

**Have high dose steroids been added?** — No →

Steroids increase the effectiveness of other anti-emetics. (mechanism unknown).

Yes ↓

Consider:
- Admission to hospice
- Ondansetron SC
- Octreotide SC
- Higher dose Methotrimeprazine
- Sedation (eg lorazepam)

# NAUSEA AND VOMITING

**What is the cause?**
Assessment (history, examination and tests) often reveals a potentially reversible cause (or causes). Treat with anti-emetics <u>simultaneously</u> with looking for and treating any underlying causes (eg infection, metabolic etc). If no cause is found it is probably due to tumour-related peptides (as yet unidentified).

**Is it large volume vomiting?**
This is usually due to malignant pyloric (high) obstruction, with projectile vomiting and often little preceding nausea. High dose steroids can reduce peri-tumour oedema and will "unblock" about 50%. A venting gastrostomy is a last resort but can stop vomiting and allow the patient to eat and drink normally (even though little is absorbed). An nasogastric tube should be a short-term measure but may allow a patient to get home. <u>Gastric stasis</u> causes reflux and heartburn as well as (<u>non</u>-projectile) vomiting and is often opioid-induced. Consider change of opioid.

**Is the nausea controlled by oral anti-emetics?**
Nausea causes gastric stasis. Oral anti-emetics may be poorly absorbed if there is nausea even without vomiting. Control nausea with IM\SC or PR drugs, and reserve oral anti-emetics for preventing recurrence.

**Which anti-emetic?**
The principle is to tailor the choice of anti-emetics to the likely cause of the nausea or vomiting. Although we are beginning to understand more about the receptor activity of these drugs, clinical practice is still largely based on experience, trial-and-error, and a limited logic:

| | |
|---|---|
| Gastrokinetic | eg metoclopramide |
| Anticholinergic | eg cyclizine |
| Antidompaminergic | eg metoclopremide, haloperidol |
| 5 HT3 | eg ondansetron |
| Broad-spectrum | eg methotrimeprazine |

30% of patients need more than one anti-emetic (and it is logical to combine drugs with different receptor activities).

**Is it due to obstruction?**
If surgery is not possible or appropriate the symptoms can be managed with a SC infusion of drugs. The aim is to abolish nausea, pain and colic. It may not be possible to abolish vomiting altogether in obstruction, but the patient can still eat and drink and most patients tolerate the occasional vomit well provided they are free of nausea (see Subcutaneous infusions).

**Is nausea or vomiting difficult to control?**
Monitor treatment by asking the patient to keep a DIARY of their symptoms, which helps analyse the pattern. It may be necessary to admit the patient for re-hydration, therapeutic trials or investigations. Quite often the symptom settles in the more secure environment of a hospice, suggesting anxiety is one component of the problem.

*See also*: Subcutaneous drugs.

# PAIN CONTROL

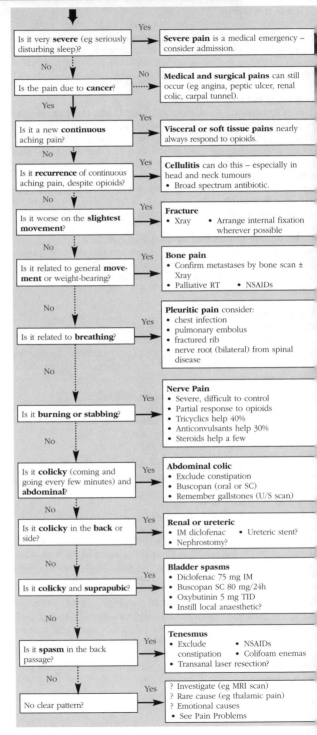

**Is it very severe (eg seriously disturbing sleep)?** — Yes → **Severe pain** is a medical emergency – consider admission.

No ↓

**Is the pain due to cancer?** — No ⋯⋯ → **Medical and surgical pains** can still occur (eg angina, peptic ulcer, renal colic, carpal tunnel).

Yes ↓

**Is it a new continuous aching pain?** — Yes → **Visceral or soft tissue pains** nearly always respond to opioids.

No ↓

**Is it recurrence of continuous aching pain, despite opioids?** — Yes → **Cellulitis** can do this – especially in head and neck tumours
• Broad spectrum antibiotic.

No ↓

**Is it worse on the slightest movement?** — Yes → **Fracture**
• Xray    • Arrange internal fixation wherever possible

No ↓

**Is it related to general movement or weight-bearing?** — Yes → **Bone pain**
• Confirm metastases by bone scan ± Xray
• Palliative RT    • NSAIDs

No ↓

**Is it related to breathing?** — Yes → **Pleuritic pain** consider:
• chest infection
• pulmonary embolus
• fractured rib
• nerve root (bilateral) from spinal disease

No ↓

**Is it burning or stabbing?** — Yes → **Nerve Pain**
• Severe, difficult to control
• Partial response to opioids
• Tricyclics help 40%
• Anticonvulsants help 30%
• Steroids help a few

No ↓

**Is it colicky (coming and going every few minutes) and abdominal?** — Yes → **Abdominal colic**
• Exclude constipation
• Buscopan (oral or SC)
• Remember gallstones (U/S scan)

No ↓

**Is it colicky in the back or side?** — Yes → **Renal or ureteric**
• IM diclofenac    • Ureteric stent?
• Nephrostomy?

No ↓

**Is it colicky and suprapubic?** — Yes → **Bladder spasms**
• Diclofenac 75 mg IM
• Buscopan SC 80 mg/24h
• Oxybutinin 5 mg TID
• Instill local anaesthetic?

No ↓

**Is it spasm in the back passage?** — Yes → **Tenesmus**
• Exclude constipation    • NSAIDs    • Colifoam enemas
• Transanal laser resection?

No ↓

**No clear pattern?** — Yes → ? Investigate (eg MRI scan)
? Rare cause (eg thalamic pain)
? Emotional causes
• See Pain Problems

**This flow-chart** is about routine methods of pain control for cancer pain. 30% of patients with cancer do not get cancer pain.

## How should I assess pain?

Most pains are diagnosed from the pattern described by the patient. Ask about:

**P** = Place?
**A** = Analgesics tried?
**R** = Relation to movement?
**T** = Timing?
**N** = Nights and sleep?
**E** = Exacerbating factors?
**R** = Relieving factors?
**S** = Severity (0–10)?

## Is it cancer pain?

Careful assessment (especially history-taking) is the key to good management. A simple example: A patient with liver metastases may have abdominal pains and may be started on morphine on the assumption that the pain is cancer pain. However the liver metastases may be pain free and the pain may be colicky pain due to constipation (which will be worsened by the morphine). It is essential to explore the pattern of each pain and to be on the look-out for non-cancer pain.

## How should I assess cancer pain?

The patient's verbal report of the pain, which usually gives a clear indication of the type of cancer pain: <u>Continuous</u> pain (visceral or soft tissue) usually responds well to morphine. Pain <u>on movement</u> (bone pain) responds poorly to morphine, but is usually controlled by radiotherapy or NSAIDs. <u>Stabbing or burning</u> pain (nerve pain) responds partially to morphine, but usually needs tricyclics or anti-convulsants as well. <u>Colicky</u> pain that comes and goes may be due to treatable constipation or may respond to an anti-spasmodic, such as Buscopan.

## Is the treatment controlling the pain?

**PAIN SCORES** are an effective and simple way to monitor pain control. The patient is asked 3 times a day to rate the severity of pain on a score of 0–10, where 0 is no pain at all and 10 is the worst pain imaginable. The scores are recorded on a chart. Uncontrolled pain needs re-assessment.

<u>See also</u> Analgesia, Fentanyl, Morphine.

# SLEEP PROBLEMS

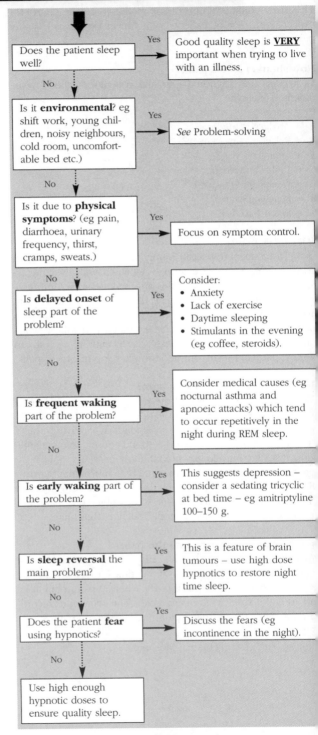

Does the patient sleep well? — **Yes** → Good quality sleep is **VERY** important when trying to live with an illness.

No

Is it **environmental**? eg shift work, young children, noisy neighbours, cold room, uncomfortable bed etc.) — **Yes** → *See* Problem-solving

No

Is it due to **physical symptoms**? (eg pain, diarrhoea, urinary frequency, thirst, cramps, sweats.) — **Yes** → Focus on symptom control.

No

Is **delayed onset** of sleep part of the problem? — **Yes** → Consider:
- Anxiety
- Lack of exercise
- Daytime sleeping
- Stimulants in the evening (eg coffee, steroids).

No

Is **frequent waking** part of the problem? — **Yes** → Consider medical causes (eg nocturnal asthma and apnoeic attacks) which tend to occur repetitively in the night during REM sleep.

No

Is **early waking** part of the problem? — **Yes** → This suggests depression – consider a sedating tricyclic at bed time – eg amitriptyline 100–150 g.

No

Is **sleep reversal** the main problem? — **Yes** → This is a feature of brain tumours – use high dose hypnotics to restore night time sleep.

No

Does the patient **fear** using hypnotics? — **Yes** → Discuss the fears (eg incontinence in the night).

No

Use high enough hypnotic doses to ensure quality sleep.

**Insomnia** is a very unpleasant experience that worsens most symptoms and if severe it becomes a medical emergency.

## Is the patient frightened of sleeping?
Many patients feel they may die in their sleep and not wake up. This responds to explanation and establishing trust so the patient can use hypnotics. If the patients have nightmares ask about what happened and how they felt. It helps to verbalise fears and it is safer to discuss fears relating to the dream rather than to dying.

## Is insomnia resistant to high dose hypnotics?
Add Chlorpromazine 25–50mg. If insomnia is severe and distressing then an IM injection of Diamorphine 2.5–5mg, Chlorpromazine 50mg Hyoscine 0.4mg guarantees 4 hours sleep for most patients.

## Which hypnotic?
Temazepam (10–60mg) suits many patients, but not all. If temazepam is too powerful choose one of the very short acting hypnotics (eg zolpidem). If temazepam has little effect consider a longer active one (eg nitrazepam).

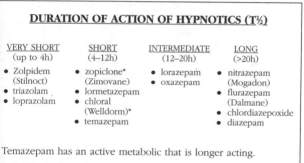

### DURATION OF ACTION OF HYPNOTICS (T½)

| VERY SHORT (up to 4h) | SHORT (4–12h) | INTERMEDIATE (12–20h) | LONG (>20h) |
|---|---|---|---|
| • Zolpidem (Stilnoct) | • zopiclone* (Zimovane) | • lorazepam | • nitrazepam (Mogadon) |
| • triazolam | • lormetazepam | • oxazepam | • flurazepam (Dalmane) |
| • loprazolam | • chloral (Welldorm)* | | • chlordiazepoxide |
| | • temazepam | | • diazepam |

Temazepam has an active metabolic that is longer acting.

\* Not benzodiazepines

## What dose of hypnotic?
The dose needed is very variable but should be high enough to be effective. Sleep is very important. The dose may need to be increased after 2–3 weeks because tolerance develops to benzodiazepines if taken regularly.

# SPINAL CORD COMPRESSION

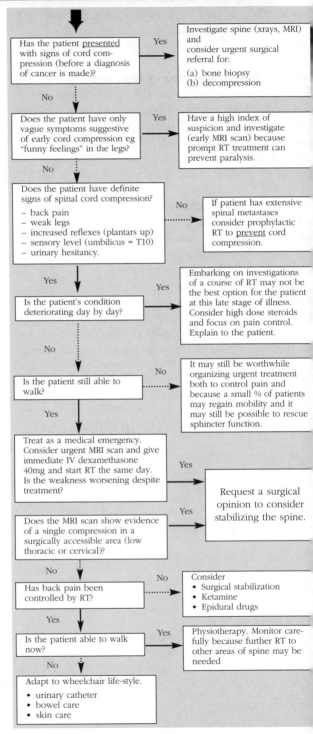

Has the patient <u>presented</u> with signs of cord compression (before a diagnosis of cancer is made)? — **Yes** → Investigate spine (xrays, MRI) and consider urgent surgical referral for:
(a) bone biopsy
(b) decompression

**No**

Does the patient have only vague symptoms suggestive of early cord compression eg "funny feelings" in the legs? — **Yes** → Have a high index of suspicion and investigate (early MRI scan) because prompt RT treatment can prevent paralysis.

**No**

Does the patient have definite signs of spinal cord compression?
– back pain
– weak legs
– increased reflexes (plantars up)
– sensory level (umbilicus = T10)
– urinary hesitancy.
— **No** → If patient has extensive spinal metastases consider prophylactic RT to <u>prevent</u> cord compression.

**Yes**

Is the patient's condition deteriorating day by day? — **Yes** → Embarking on investigations of a course of RT may not be the best option for the patient at this late stage of illness. Consider high dose steroids and focus on pain control. Explain to the patient.

**No**

Is the patient still able to walk? — **No** → It may still be worthwhile organizing urgent treatment both to control pain and because a small % of patients may regain mobility and it may still be possible to rescue sphincter function.

**Yes**

Treat as a medical emergency. Consider urgent MRI scan and give immediate IV dexamethasone 40mg and start RT the same day. Is the weakness worsening despite treatment? — **Yes** → Request a surgical opinion to consider stabilizing the spine.

Does the MRI scan show evidence of a single compression in a surgically accessible area (low thoracic or cervical)? — **Yes** → Request a surgical opinion to consider stabilizing the spine.

**No**

Has back pain been controlled by RT? — **No** → Consider
• Surgical stabilization
• Ketamine
• Epidural drugs

**Yes**

Is the patient able to walk now? — **Yes** → Physiotherapy. Monitor carefully because further RT to other areas of spine may be needed

**No**

Adapt to wheelchair life-style.
• urinary catheter
• bowel care
• skin care

# SPINAL CORD COMPRESSION

## Is cord compression common?

10% of patients with spinal metastases develop cord compression during the course of their illness. It is usually a complication of far advanced disease, but 10–20% of these patients survive for 12 months. Cord compression may rarely occur as a presenting symptom, before the diagnosis of cancer is known.

## Is this early cord compression?

The complaint of "funny feelings" in both legs should be taken very seriously, especially if there is a new thoracic spinal pain. Urgent MRI scan is indicated – even if the other signs of cord compression are not obvious. Cord compression usually occurs in the thoracic region (70)%, but may occur in the lumbosacral region (20%) or the cervical spine (10%). Lung, breast, prostate are the commonest causes.

## What are the signs of cord compression?

If both legs are weak, or feel "funny" and the reflexes are brisk, and the plantar reflexes are upgoing then a cord compression is highly likely. 90% of patients will have back pain. Loss of sensation below a certain level (a "sensory level") occurs usually somewhere between nipples (T4) and the umbilicus (T10) – but may not be obvious for the first 24 hours. Urinary hesitancy is usually a late feature.

## Is the patient still walking?

If the patient is still walking, emergency treatment gives a 1 in 3 chance of retaining leg strength. Act quickly – give immediate IV steroids and aim to start radiotherapy treatment within 24 hours.

## Does the patient have a short prognosis?

If a patient has established cord compression and probably only has a short prognosis (eg week-by-week deterioration) it may not be in their best interests to embark on a course of radiotherapy. Discuss the options with the patient, if possible. A single treatment of radiotherapy to the spine may be adequate for pain control.

## Have we set realistic short-term goals for rehabilitation?

Once the patient is paraplegic, usually with double incontinence (and impotence in men). Focus on breaking the bad news that recovery will probably not occur (rather than waiting inappropriately for strength to return). The focus of management shifts to helping the patient (and family) adjust to wheel-chair mobility and to managing the problems of paraplegia (skin and bowel care, managing a catheter, wheel-chair access to home etc). Setting realistic short-term goals is the key to good management.

# STEROIDS

Might steroids improve this symptom?

**No** ....... About 40% of hospice patients benefit from a course of steroids at some point.

**Yes** ↓

Have steroids already been tried for this problem?

**Yes** → The first course of steroids usually gives the best response for symptom control.

**No** ↓

Is the patient willing to try steroids?

**No** ....... Some patients are frightened of the side-effects of steroids, having seen other people have side-effects – especially weight gain or facial swelling.

**Yes** ↓

Is the prognosis likely to be more than 3 months?

**Yes** → There is more likelihood of developing distressing side-effects (facial swelling) if steroids are used for more than a few weeks – consider postponing steroid use or consider megestrol 160mg OD as an alternative for anorexia.

**No** ↓

Is the patient diabetic?

**Yes** → Steroids increase blood glucose. Non-insulin dependent diabetics may need to start insulin (discuss this before starting steroids) and those on insulin will probably need to increase their dose of insulin.

**No** ↓

Does the patient take NSAIDS or have a history of peptic ulcer?

**Yes** → The risk of ulceration and perforation is increased. Give gastro-protective therapy – eg omeprazole 20mg OD.

**No** ↓

Does the patient have a history of insomnia, agitation or paranoia?

**Yes** → Steroids can cause insomnia (therefore give early in the day) and can worsen agitation – an effective option sometimes is to give haloperidol 3–5mg daily or BD with the steroids.

**No** ↓

Give a 7 day course of steroids. Has the symptom improved?

**No** ....... Stop steroids if no benefit occurs. Consider other treatments.

**Yes** ↓

Issue Steroid Card. Reduce dose very gradually (eg 2mg per week) to try to maintain improvement but reduce the risk of long-term steroid side-effects.

→ Monitor for:
• oral thrush
• ankle oedema
• diabetes
• gastric problems

## Who needs steroids?

50% of cancer patients benefit from steroids at some time.

## What is the correct dose?

Dexamethasone is preferred because it has less miner-alo-corticoid activity than prednisolone. The aim is to improve symptoms then to reduce rapidly to the lowest effective dose and to discontinue if there is no benefit.

| What dose of dexamethasone? | |
|---|---|
| Dose | Indication |
| *2 – 4 mg* | Anorexia, fatigue |
| *8 – 12 mg* | To decrease tumour oedema |
| *16 – 32 mg* | Raised ICP, cord compression |

## Should antifungals be started?

Oral thrush is such a common complication in patients on steroids that prophylacticd Nystatin 1 ml QDS is sometimes advised routinely for <u>all</u> patients starting steroids.

## Who needs gastro-protection?

About 20% of patients on steroids need gastro-protection. The risk of peptic ulceration on steroids is dou-bled from 1 to 2% but this means 98% are not at increased risk. Gastro-protection is indicated if a patient is on concurrent NSAID's, has had a total dose above 140 mg of Dexamethasone or has a previous history of peptic ulceration, (all of which increase the risk of ulceration or perforation). Misoprostol is the most effective treatment to protect against NSAID's otherwise ranitidine or omeprazole can be used.

## How are steroids stopped?

Steroids can be stopped immediately if the patient has been on less than 6mg of Dexamethazone for less than 3 weeks (or if the patient is in the last few days of life). In other patients steroids should be stopped gradually because adrenal surpression will have occurred. The physiological dose is Dexamethasone 1 mg (Prednisolone 7 mg ) so a sensible regime is to use Prednisolone 5 mg daily and reduce by 1 mg every 3 days finishing with 1 mg alternate days for a week.

## WHICH DRUGS FOR SC INFUSION?

| DRUG AMPOULES | STARTING DOSE PER 24 HOUR | MAIN USE | NOTES |
|---|---|---|---|
| **Diamorphine** 10,30,100,500 mg | 15 mg | Pain | These drugs are often mixed together in combinations of 2, 3 (and sometimes 4) with good effect. This is established good practice but outside the licensing indications for most of the drugs. Definitive data on their compatibilities is still lacking. Seek advice if unsure which drugs to use. |
| **Cyclizine** 50 mg/1 ml | 100 mg | Sickness | |
| **Metoclopramide** 10 mg/2 ml | 30 mg | Sickness | |
| **Haloperidol** 5 mg/1 ml | 2.5 mg | Drug-induced nausea | |
| **Methotrime- prazine** 25 mg/1 ml | 12.5 mg | Broad-spectrum powerful anti-emetic | |
| **Midazolam** 10 mg/2 ml | 10 mg | Agitation Anti-convulsant | |
| **Hyoscine hydrobromide** 0.4 mg/1 ml 0.6 mg/1 ml | 1.2 mg | Bubbling | |
| **Buscopan (hyoscine butylbromide)** 20 mg/1 ml | 40 mg | Colic | |
| **Dexamethasone** 4 mg/1 ml | 4 mg | Reduces peri tumour oedema | Add last & slowly. Does not mix with cylizine |
| **Octreotide** 100 mcg/1 ml 500 mcg/1 ml | 100 mcg | Reduces gastro-intestinal secretions | Does not mix with cyclizine or dexamethasone |
| **Ketamine** 500 mg/5 ml | 100 mg | Difficult pain problems | Strong non-opioid. Mixes with diamorphine, haloperidol or midazolam. Dose range 100–600 mg per 24 hour. |
| **Phenobarbitone** 200 mg/1 ml | 200 mg | Anti-convulsant | Use separate pump |
| **Diclofenac** 75 mg/3 ml | 150 mg | Severe bone pain | • Use separate pump • Avoid in renal failure |
| **Ondansetron** 2 mg/1 ml | 8 mg | Chemotherapy induced nausea | Use separate pump. |
| **Hyaluronidase** 1500 units/ ampoule | 1500 units | Dispersal of SC fluids. (May also decrease inflammation at injection site | Prime the line with it. Not if allergy or asthma. |

## Which drugs can be given subcutaneously?

Many drugs are effective via a subcutaneous infusion. Common combinations include diamorphine, cyclizine and Buscopan (eg in malignant intestinal obstruction) or diamorhine, midazolam and hyoscine (eg in the terminal phase). The number of drugs being given by the SC route is steadily increasing with experience.

## Which drugs can be combined?

Which drugs are combined is based on clinical experience of what works. Many drugs will mix together without precipitation and are clinically effective (although it remains unknown whether partial inactivation is occurring). Drugs which tend to precipitate with other drugs are cyclizine and dexamethasone – if precipitation in a mixture is occurring it is often due to one of these drugs. Certain drugs need to be given in a separate syringe pump, eg diclofenac, phenobarbitone.

## Are the drugs licensed for this use?

In Palliative Medicine about 15% of prescriptions are for unlicensed indications.

Many drugs given by the SC route are not licensed for use in this way. The Medicines Act of 1968 permit the use of unlicensed medicines, or licensed drugs for unlicensed purposes provided the prescriber is acting in concordance with past practice of others in the field. Legally the doctor must be aware of the licence status of the drug and as with all prescribing, should use reasonable skill and care, and normally have the patient's informed consent – eg it should have been explained carefully first.

## What if a skin reaction occurs?

Skin reactions can occur especially with cyclizine and methotrimeprazine and the site then needs changing daily. Increasing the dilution (use a 30cc syringe) can help. Some patients are allergic to the metal in the butterfly – use a plastic cannula. Non–sterile technique can result in abscesses.

# TERMINAL PHASE

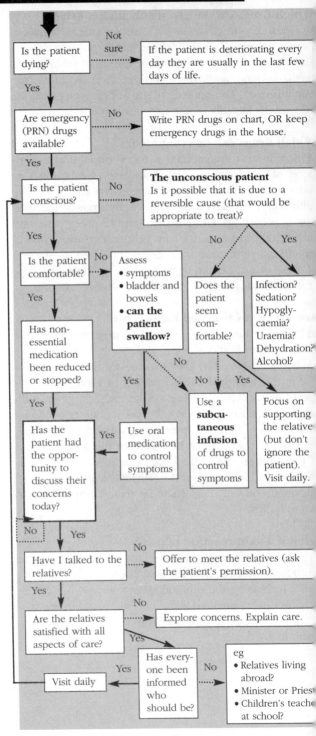

**Is the patient dying?** — Not sure ⟶ If the patient is deteriorating every day they are usually in the last few days of life.

Yes ↓

**Are emergency (PRN) drugs available?** — No ⟶ Write PRN drugs on chart, OR keep emergency drugs in the house.

Yes ↓

**Is the patient conscious?** — No ⟶ **The unconscious patient** Is it possible that it is due to a reversible cause (that would be appropriate to treat)?

No ↓    Yes ⟶ Infection? Sedation? Hypoglycaemia? Uraemia? Dehydration? Alcohol?

Yes ↓

**Is the patient comfortable?** — No ⟶ Assess
- symptoms
- bladder and bowels
- **can the patient swallow?**

Does the patient seem comfortable?

Yes ↓

**Has non-essential medication been reduced or stopped?**

No ⟶ Use a **subcutaneous infusion** of drugs to control symptoms

Yes ⟶ Focus on supporting the relative (but don't ignore the patient). Visit daily.

Swallow Yes ⟶ Use oral medication to control symptoms

Yes ↓

**Has the patient had the opportunity to discuss their concerns today?**

No ↓    Yes ↓

**Have I talked to the relatives?** — No ⟶ Offer to meet the relatives (ask the patient's permission).

Yes ↓

**Are the relatives satisfied with all aspects of care?** — No ⟶ Explore concerns. Explain care.

Yes ↓

**Has everyone been informed who should be?** — No ⟶ eg
- Relatives living abroad?
- Minister or Priest
- Children's teacher at school?

Yes ⟶ Visit daily

## Is the patient dying?

The diagnosis of "dying" is VERY important because it changes medical decision-making. Once a patient is diagnosed as dying:

- investigations become irrelevant
- aiming to prolong life becomes irrelevant
- patient comfort takes priority
- increased support for the family is needed

If the patient has a progressive incurable disease, if reversible causes of deterioration have been excluded (eg infection hypercalcaemia) and if they are very weak and drowsy and getting weaker every day, then they are dying.

## What is the role of the doctor?

The doctor continues to have a key role when a patient is dying (and some doctors seem to be unaware of this):

- visit daily
- liaise with nursing team
- asses patient's comfort
- review medication
- support the relatives (see Family Meetings)

Families are always very grateful for the skilled medical supervision of their dying relative.

## How do I monitor an unconscious patient?

Visit daily, liaise with the nursing team about nursing care (eye care, mouth care regular timing, catheter care, bowel care). Monitor medication and assess level of consciousness, using EYELID FLICKER TEST. When the eyelid is touched in deeply unconscious patients there is no effect. Relatives find it reassuring when the doctor talks to a patient even when unconscious (eg "It is Dr Kaye, Michael, I am just going to touch your eyelid and test a reflex".)

## What medication is used?

A subcutaneous infusion of drugs is very helpful if the patients can no longer swallow. A common combination is diamorphine (for pain or dyspnoea), hyoscine (to dry up respiratory secretions and control the terminal bubbling) and midazolam if there is any terminal agitation.

| | |
|---|---|
| Diamorphine | mg\24hr (dose = 50% oral morphine\24hr) |
| Hyoscine | 0.8–1.6 mg\24hr |
| Midazolam | 10–60 mg\24hr |

## How can the patient be protected from too many visitors?

Many dying patients have a dilemma about visitors, wanting the support but getting exhausted by TOO MANY (well meaning) VISITORS – consider a "medical edict" to set limits and suggest a visiting rota (so visitors can also get some rest).

*See also* Dehydration, Subcutaneous drugs.